DIY Body Detox Natural Rituals!

The DIY Natural Homemade Remedy for Lifelong Beauty, Wellness and All-Natural Life!

Dr. Jane Wells

INTRODUCTION

Body cleanse detox is the discussion of the period. Indeed, it is!

It has nearly become A-recorded like practice to join this action in your day by day lives. So, you check out yourself and the word hits your ear-DETOX!

The responses are blended individuals catching wind of it, interestingly are captivated by it and are excited about discovering more about it. Individuals previously rehearsing it are enthusiastic about conveying data about it. Detox has been accumulating enormous exposure in recent years with everything taken into account, which is solid indeed.

Your body resembles your home, and you should realize it as you know yourself. For appropriate everyday working of the body, various cycles inside the body should be completed.

For this to occur, the body parts which play out these capacities should be all together.

This is the place where detox comes into the picture. Natural functions such as discharging waste from the body are an interaction completed by different parts of your body like the liver, kidneys, skin, and so forth; these need ordinary upkeep and detox assists you with doing as such.

They need upkeep because they are consistently intentionally or accidentally presented to hazardous and destructive components that are amazingly hurtful. Air just as water contamination are on the ascent and like this indirectly affect our body frameworks. Lungs are defenseless against smoke, whether it is being discharged as a vapor because of fuel ignition in vehicles or the toxins from smoking tobacco biting and cigarette smoking.

Dietary examples are additionally evolving radically. Manures and insect poisons and pesticides that are initially intended to furnish us with solid soil products are discovering their direction into our bodies through food varieties on which they have been showered and causing serious infections, all things being equal. Meat as pork, ham, and steak, chicken is sold with drugs for an overhauled quality.

This load of toxic and hurtful poisons are influencing our excretory framework massively. The expanded shortcoming is being noticed for the most part since the time these progressions have begun occurring.

The effects are there for you to see with yourselves own eyes. There is expanded aggravation, swelling of the body, dormancy, bluntness of the skin, parchedness, and expansion in the bodyweight; there is a monstrous danger of succumbing to sicknesses like joint pain and diabetes malignancies, heart illnesses, and the rundown goes on.

Avoidance is superior to fix. It is smart to take estimates at first, so you are not liable to bother about your body. Be that as it may, it can still be corrected. Even get-togethers are analyzed, and there are odds of recovery. Be that as it may, the demonstration should happen soon.

Detox. Albeit sluggish, however, a definite one at that assists you with keeping up with your body at the most flawless level. You could alter your detox modules as per your body needs and take a pick. You could browse an assortment of projects like the one that permits just new products of the soil juices or the one that doesn't allow prepared food, or the one wherein supplement are not needed. The aggregate point of this load of modules is only one to assist you in disposing all gathered noxious substances.

CHAPTER 1

Why DIY Body Detox

Data are abundant out there about Detox - it very well may be confounding and hard to tell what is the best thing to do. I will make a valiant effort to give you straightforward rules that will help you track down the best intend to suit you and your way of life.

The one thing you know is that you're not feeling your best, and you need to take care of business. This is a great beginning, and via looking for this data, you are venturing out to working on your wellbeing, ideally for all time. Useful for you - in a real sense!

We as a whole realize when we're feeling poisonous - we can look puffy, feel drained and impassive, possibly somewhat discouraged, and as though everything is somewhat of a battle. We may even experience a blockage, skin issues, throbbing joints, and uneasiness.

For What Reason Do We Need to Detox?

Regularly - in a sound and indigenous habitat - our bodies are more than equipped for detoxing themselves, keeping each cell perfect and functioning as it ought to keep you stimulated and loaded with wellbeing and strength.

Shockingly the world we live in is presently not beneficial and regular. We are continually besieged with unpredictable and handled synthetic substances that our bodies find hard to use successfully. These toxins are in our air, water, and food, just as we use them in beautifiers and family cleaning items. These poisons can develop in the body and cause harm to tissues and cells.

Thus, the measure of poisons that our organic entity needs to manage each day can overpower our innate capacity to scrub. A lot is coming in for our frameworks to have the opportunity and energy to sort it into classifications and discard it all securely. It's somewhat similar to the neighborhood Council dump - they need to close the doors when they are excessively occupied with making sure they can make up for lost time and wipe out the avoids prepared for the following part of waste to show up! The thing that detoxing is - it ends the entryways and not letting any longer garbage in until you've managed the build-up!

It is the stopping of processing that empowers the body to have the opportunity to clean itself. The less you digest, the more poisons you'll have the option to deliver.

Will I Lose Weight?

Getting thinner is one of the principal motivating forces for individuals to do a Detox. In all actuality, they regularly find that getting thinner is only a special reward instead of the principal advantage. The expansion in essentialness and general energy for your life will bring about a difference in diet and life. This will carry an inside and out progress in wellbeing on all levels that, it just so happens, incorporates being a good weight!

Which Detox is Best For You?

Suppose this is your first Detox, it is best to begin with, a multi-day plan, so it's safe and straightforward for you to do. You can go from that point to a more extended program or a directed, private retreat to settle the score more, longer enduring advantages.

You can expand the aftereffects of the Detox hugely by planning for it as long as you can progress over time. By eliminating your admission of poisons before your multi-day Detox, you will decrease the detox indications and increment the viability of your purge.

Getting ready for Your Cleanse

Make this attempt to keep away from the accompanying for at least seven days before you start. Caffeine, liquor, sugar, cigarettes, fake sugars, and refined, prepared food sources. Assuming you need to eat meat, then, at that point, attempt and purchase natural meat from a neighborhood source. Modest meat can contains steroids, chemicals, and anti-infection agents. I enthusiastically suggest shopping in your neighborhood wellbeing food shop instead of the general store as it is a lot simpler to discover the food sources you need and some you didn't know existed!

Attempt to eat like a creature! Get ready food varieties that seem as though they did when they were developing. Bunches of organic products, vegetables, entire grains, and heartbeats are a superb and practical wellspring of essential supplements - without the poisons.

Taste a lot of water for the day - somewhere around eight glasses alongside homegrown and organic product teas. This will assist with flushing the poisons out of your body and decrease any detox side effects you may be having. These manifestations can incorporate cerebral pains, hurting, sluggishness, yearnings, and even emotional episodes.

These manifestations emerge because the body delivers an excessive number of poisons for the liver to process and deliver. To help the liver, you could attempt an enhancement or homegrown color that upholds the liver, like Dandelion or Milk Thistle. You can likewise purchase great quality Detox tea (generally at your neighborhood wellbeing food shop or from a botanist); this can likewise help the liver during your detox.

During the week before your scrub, have a go at giving your liver and gallbladder a lift by taking two tablespoons of good quality olive oil blended in with two tablespoons of lemon juice. Do this each day first thing for five days.

Blending a spoon of nectar in with juice vinegar additionally has a detoxifying, re-adjusting influence on the liver.

CHAPTER 2

Detoxing in case You're Busy

On the off chance that you need to continue with your regular daily schedule while detoxing, I suggest a mono diet. This permits you to continue taking in energy without the body needing to endeavor to process the food.

1. In the colder time of year, I would suggest an earthy-colored rice purge. This is so basic and modest to do. Purchase an amount of natural, short-grain earthy colored rice, cook for 45 minutes in twofold the measure of water to rice and eat only that for three days. Try not to add salt or preparing to keep it as simple to process as could be expected.

2. In the spring or summer, three days of eating only natural grapes is a decent method to keep your glucose step up while permitting a profound and careful spring clean.

You can expand the advantage of both these weight control plans by pressing a new lemon into a glass of water in the first part of the day.

The advantages of the mono-diet are that it is not difficult to get ready and convey the food you need with you, and it is straightforward to do.

Detoxing if You Have More Time

On the off chance that you're discovering the Detox too troublesome, increment the assortment of the food you're eating. The members just have weakened juices for six days on the retreat - this empowers a deep and powerful scrub. Just by giving somebody a pure, undiluted juice, we can significantly sluggish the impacts of their Detox.

Assuming you need to have a deep detox, then, at that point, stick to juices - if this is too hard, then add servings of mixed greens, entire organic product, seeds, and some straightforward prepared food. This will decrease the indications and the power of the purge. Continuously pay attention to your body's needs (desires can be deluding - the body doesn't require chocolate and coffee!!).

Again - start the day with lemon juice in water. Drink just water and natural teas during the day.

If you have a juicer, purchase determination of new, natural vegetables (ideally privately developed) and squeeze these in the blend to make an assortment of delightful, nutritious beverages. Additionally, by adding a superfood, for example, spirulina, you can make your juices much more nutritious and alkalizing to the body. You can add root ginger to your juices for a warming and delicious option.

You can either have squeezes and organic products or make plates of mixed greens with a combination of crude vegetables. Ground beetroot, carrot, and cabbage can add mass and goodness. Beetroot is beneficial for the liver. You can add seeds and grew beats (promptly accessible from wellbeing food shops or simple to grow at home) and dress with a virus squeezed olive oil and lemon juice or apple juice vinegar.

Assuming you need to incorporate prepared food, then, at that point, daintily steam vegetables and have with a modest quantity of earthy colored rice or quinoa dressed with olive oil, a little tamari (wheat-free soya sauce), or a tahini dressing which can be made with a spoonful of tahini (back to the wellbeing food shop) blended bit by bit with some water to make it a smooth, runny consistency. Add ginger and tamari, lemon, or juice vinegar if you genuinely need more flavor.

Attempt to eat all your food gradually and modestly and make sure to take half an hour of mild exercise ordinary.

A Supervised Detox

At a Detox Retreat, the staff can be sure that each member gets precisely what they, by and by, need. They give supplements the juices that are explicitly intended to upgrade the purging project. They decrease hunger, clean the entrail, gather the delivered poisons (to keep them from being re-retained), and extricate old matter put away in the digestive organs. Juices are given and possibly a mineral stock each day, and they will ideally have a Detox master close by to encourage and uphold every person.

Withdraws, as a rule, additionally give colonic water system, either gravity or Coleman hardware in every washroom so members can have self-controlled colonics or managed automated colonics. The job of the colonic is to accelerate the purging cycle by, in a real sense washing the poisons and old matter out of the entrail. All the undesirable waste that is delivered into the entrail is washed clean away by this primary cycle. It feels astounding!

A decent Detox Retreat will offer passionate and commonsense help and guidance, back rub, and mending treatments just as talks and dietary data to take into your day-by-day life. Light exercise can be given by yoga and directed strolls just as the spa and rec center offices. Just so the otherworldly side isn't left out, you might have directed contemplations to begin the day.

The Detox Retreat is there for individuals who would prefer not to detox at home and feel that they would profit with more help and direction. Those individuals who have different medical problems could profit with a more drawn-out and more profound purge.

Chapter 3

Medical advantages of Lemon Water

How about we be completely clear. Lemon water without help from anyone else isn't a detox. Lemon water helps our bodies during the time spent flushing the poisons out and reestablishing the liver. However, to flush your framework, you will likewise require fiber, since let's be honest, lemons, while high in Vitamin C, are not high in fiber. The present blog centers around the "additional items" to hold onto your consideration while likewise taking your water toasting to a higher level. Appreciate!

Drinking Lemon Water benefits

Stomach-related wellbeing, Weight misfortune, practice execution, emotional wellness, advanced hydration, an incredible wellspring of Vitamin C, balances body pH against maturing properties, detoxes liver, urinary plot scrub, and a straightforward and financially savvy approach to improve wellbeing.

Step by step instructions to Make Lemon Water

Assuming you need to see the wellbeing and health advantages of drinking lemon water, you should devour it consistently. Likewise, utilize new lemons.

Fixings

1/2 lemon

1/2 cup cold water

1/2 cup heated water

Directions

In the glass, crush lemon juice into 1 cup of cold water. Mix and drink while warm.

What's in Store

In the advanced world, our bodies are under steady attack from different poisons; Toxins we ingest through food and drink, those found in our current circumstance, to those made as a result inside our body.

The liver is the purifying place of this load of poisons, yet sometimes it's capacity to detox productively becomes debilitated because of consistent stacking.

When these poisons can presently don't be disposed of, they are put away as muscle to fat ratio to be managed some time in the future. Except if you give your body the opportunity, it needs to deal with these poisons out of your body; they'll develop, adding to a condition called greasy liver.

By doing a detox or limiting the poisons your body needs to measure, you give your liver the space it needs to begin handling these poisons once more. When prepared, they are delivered into the lymphatic framework, kidneys, and blood to be killed. Over the top poisons left long enough in the body can introduce an entire host of issues and wellbeing concerns.

In this blog, we'll be taking a gander at the advantages of detoxing, food sources that typically assist your body with detoxing, and what is going on inside your body that causes the 'detox impact,' or 'mending emergency.'

All in all, why Detox?

Help re-balance the body and fix the harm.

Remove natural poisons that have developed in your body.

Diminish indications of migraines, hurts, aggravation, skin break out, and expanded muscle to fat ratio.

Diminish your reliance on energizers like sugar, caffeine, and refined carbs.

What's Happening Inside Your Body when Detoxing?

1. The overall clarification

Everyone will begin a detox for various reasons and from various degrees of harmfulness. When discussing an overall clarification, recall that everybody's bodies are one of a kind. Therefore, every one of us will have various encounters when detoxing and show various manifestations.

"When in doubt, the more poisonous the body is, or the more long stretches of helpless propensities gathered, the more extreme the mending emergency will be."

When beginning a detox, you may see a transitory deteriorating of any current manifestations you have. This is typical and happens as the body gets out the 'muck.' This is a characteristic piece of the body's interaction of recuperating itself using the end of poisons collected inside your cells.

While this is usually known as a 'detox response,' we like to consider this 'a recuperating emergency's or 'mending response .' It is an essential abhorrent where you feel more terrible several days before you feel much improved.

Mending emergency or 'recuperating response,' is vital to feeling awful several days before you feel much improved.

The poisons being ousted from your body during this cycle may have been caught in the phones (or liver and gallbladder) for quite a long time (here and there, even many years). When in doubt, the more poisonous the body is, or the more prolonged periods of helpless propensities amassed, the more extraordinary the recuperating emergency will be. The disposal organs (lungs, skin, liver, kidneys) consolidate together to wipe out side-effects however can be overpowered by the interaction.

Recall that a recuperating emergency is just brief, and you are on the way to recharged wellbeing. Even though amending an emergency is awkward, it is a decent sign that the body is attempting to recuperate itself and typically lasts between 2 - 5 days.

On the off chance that you have any worries or questions, kindly call us on 0800 52 54 52, and, in case you're not feeling great under any condition during a detox, it is best to check in with your GP in every case.

2. During a sugar detox

On the off chance that you've at any point taken a stab at lessening your admission of sugar, you'll be exceptionally mindful of exactly how troublesome sugar is to cut pure and straightforward. Generally alluded to as "sugar withdrawals," this is your body's method of detoxing its reliance on using sugar to make energy.

During the sugar detox measure, many things are changing, and your body now needs to go to the additional exertion of separating fats to deliver energy. This resembles a muscle in the manner it should be prepared, and over the long run, it can become more grounded and do this quicker and more effectively. In any case, meanwhile, you'll experience detox manifestations, and you may see expanded weakness.

Likewise, when you eat a ton of sugar, your body utilizes the subsequent insulin spike to cause synapses you need to feel better. When you lessen your sugar consumption, your body needs to work more enthusiastically to make these synapses. This can cause migraines and violent, passionate swings as your body figures out how to change.

If you are hoping to lessen the measure of sugar you burn through; I suggest perusing our blog, six hints for decreasing sugar effectively and tenderly to limit the detox impact.

3. During a liquor detox

Liquor is sugar. You're not going to encounter a detox impact from liquor except if you are a drunkard and you've developed a reliance on this substance. The detox impact you will gain insight into in the present circumstance will be connected to the synapses segment we discussed in the sugar detox model above.

On the off chance that you appreciate liquor yet might want to find out about what liquor is meaning for your wellbeing, the sum you ought to drink or the best kinds to drink, have a perused of my new blog entry, 'what liquor means for your wellbeing.'

4. During a caffeine detox

Caffeine's impact on our body – and particularly on our mind – is exceptionally muddled. Caffeine chokes veins in your cerebrum and, along these lines, lessens the bloodstream. When you decrease your caffeine consumption, you're expanding the bloodstream to your mind, making your torment receptors more touchy and causes the exemplary 'caffeine cerebral pain' you experience.

Chapter 4

Normal approaches to detox

1. **Eat loads of cruciferous vegetables:** These are incredibly high in sulforaphane, which is expected to change over poisons into non-harmful material for the end—for instance, broccoli, Brussel fledglings, and kale.

2. **Eat your mixed greens:** These give valuable fiber, alkalize the body, and help to decrease irritation. Model: Spinach, silver beet, and arugula.

3. **Flaxseed oil:** As a fundamental unsaturated fat, flaxseed oil is extraordinary for raising digestion, drawing in, and restricting to oil-solvent poisons that get stopped in the liver, doing them of the framework. The fundamental unsaturated fats in flaxseed oil can likewise invigorate bile creation, which is essential for fat digestion and flushing the gallbladder.

4. **Flavors and spices**: Thermogenic flavors like ginger, cayenne, mustard, and cinnamon give bunches of flavor and raise internal heat level and launch digestion. Spices like parsley, coriander, fennel, and anise, are known for their diuretic properties to flush poisons from the body.

5. **Milk Thistle:** This can assist with expanding liver chemical creation and fix harmed liver tissue.

6. **Dandelion Root:** This and different sharp flavoring are utilized to develop processing further and decrease poison stacks discharging to the liver. Dandelion contains supplements that have been displayed to animate the liver to create bile to ship off the gallbladder and contract the gallbladder to deliver put away bile, expanding fat digestion.

7. Drink Weakened, Unsweetened Cranberry Juice: Cranberry is a significant diuretic and targets water maintenance for detoxification. Arbutin, the dynamic fixing in cranberry, pulls out the water put away in fat to be discharged by the kidneys. Cranberries are likewise loaded up with emulsifying catalysts to assist with processing fatty globules in the lymphatic framework. Since the cranberry is loaded with flavonoids, it can likewise further develop cellulite by working on the connective tissue's strength and trustworthiness and help keep the lymphatic framework working efficiently.

8. Lemon Water: This aids bile arrangement and supports energy creation through the citrus extract cycle, fundamental for fat digestion and to assist with recovering the liver. Lemon water likewise elevates peristalsis to control solid discharges and to keep the waste rushing through the stomach-related parcel for disposal.

Chapter 5

What Is The Best Beverage To Flush Your Framework?

Detox beverages may incorporate lemon, mint, cucumber, aloe vera, chia seeds, and different food sources.

Consistently, we witness another trend or idea thinking of different boosting wellbeing cases or expanding life span. Albeit rehearsed in different structures for quite a long time, detoxification or detox diet and systems have become mainstream of late. Detox counts calories guarantee that they eliminate "poisons" from the body and work on your general wellbeing. The "poisons" as referenced in these eating regimens are the principal offenders that cause medical affliction and different issues like a throbbing painfulness, going bald, skin inflammation, heftiness, dull and dry skin, joint torment, and laziness. These "poisons" incorporate different natural contaminations, pesticides, synthetic substances utilized in cultivating, food added substances, metabolic squanders delivered in the body, and different microorganisms and their metabolic items. Albeit some simple-to-make food sources and beverages guarantee to "tidy up" our "framework," do they "truly" help? There is restricted logical proof accessible to help that we "truly" need such outside detox to keep up with our bodies' strength. Our bodies have their in-assembled detoxification framework that incorporates the liver, kidneys, platelets, and antibodies. We needn't bother with any beverages or uncommon food varieties to dispose of poisons. A sound fiber-rich eating routine, regular exercise, sufficient rest, and a lot of water are adequate to keep us solid.

Detox drinks contain different leafy foods juices and, in this manner, can give different supplements. They are, nonetheless, inadequate in protein and calories. This may cause you to feel depleted or powerless. They can likewise bring down your metabolic rate since they may keep your body from calories. Most detox drinks go about as diuretics (increment your pee yield) or purgatives (increment defecations). Expanded pee yield can cause drying out, which might be seen as weight reduction. This weight reduction is brief and returns when you begin eating a customary eating routine.

Albeit different beverages might be professed to detox your body, it is shrewd to counsel a certified nutritionist or specialist before attempting them. A portion of the top beverages that case to flush your framework and detox your body incorporates

Lemon Detox Drink

Lemon is quite possibly the most well-known and staple element of detox drinks. It is plentiful in nutrient C and different cell reinforcements. It helps fabricate invulnerability and keeps the gums, bones, and skin sound. Crush a few lemons into a liter of water. You may add a touch of pink salt for the taste of it. Mesh some ginger into the lemon water and drink it. Nutrient C is heat-delicate, so ensure the water isn't hot.

Mint and cucumber detox drink: This detox drink is professed to be incredible for overseeing weight and keeping up with liquid and mineral equilibrium in the body.

Setting It Up

- Wash and strip two cucumbers and cut them into flimsy pieces.
- Wash some mint leaves and leave them up finely.
- Take a lemon and cut it into meager cuts.

- Take a wide-mouth glass jug or container and add the cut cucumber, lemon, and mint pass on to it.
- Fill it with water and some ice and refrigerate for 30 minutes to 60 minutes.
- Remove the jug from the fridge, shake it well and drink the water in taste for the day.

Coconut Water Detox Drink

This is a fast and straightforward beverage to plan. Take a glass of coconut water, add some cleaved mint to it and crush a large portion of lime into it. This is a refreshing beverage thought about proper for your skin and hair.

Chia Seed And Aloe Vera Detox Drink

Take a liter of water in a container and add a large portion of some aloe vera juice and one teaspoonful of chia seeds to it.

Allow it to rest for 10 minutes.

Press a large portion of a lemon into it, blend well and drink.

Chia seeds are sans gluten and are a decent wellspring of cancer prevention agents and calcium. They assist with directing hunger and are astounding for weight the executives.

Chapter 6

Whole Body Detox: 9 Ways To Rejuvenate Your Body

Numerous food varieties plentiful in nutrients and cell reinforcements can help your body's innate capacity to scrub and detoxify itself. Look at these nine food sources that you can add to your plate to help you feel much improved:

Feeling slow of late? Numerous food sources plentiful in nutrients and cell reinforcements can help your body's inherent capacity to scrub and detoxify itself. Not exclusively can these food varieties help your body eliminate poisons? However, they additionally give supplements that you need to lead a happy and solid life. Look at these nine food sources that you can add to your plate to help you feel much improved:

Asparagus

Asparagus contains glutathione, a notable cancer prevention agent that advances detoxification. It is also a decent wellspring of fiber, folate, iron, and nutrients A, C, E, and K, just as beneficial to those with hypertension. Asparagus is additionally known to help the kidney and bladder scrub itself.

Broccoli

Broccoli contains sulforaphane, which is extraordinary for warding off irresistible cells in our bodies. Eating broccoli likewise helps your body ward off malignancy initiating synthetic substances and lifts the liver's capacity to clear awful synthetic compounds from our bodies.

Grapefruit

Grapefruit is stacked with supplements including nutrients A, C, and B1, just as pantothenic corrosive, fiber, potassium, and biotin. Catalysts found in grapefruit may likewise separate the fat in your body to assist with advancing weight reduction. If it's not too much trouble, note that grapefruit may interface for specific prescriptions, so you ought to talk with your essential consideration supplier before expanding your grapefruit admission.

Avocado

Avocados are stacked with cell reinforcements that assist your body with removing unsafe poisons. A supplement dense food, avocados contain around 20 different nutrients and minerals that diminish the danger of weight, diabetes, and coronary illness.

Kale

What's the fight over kale? Loaded with amino acids that assist with keeping your psyche sharp, kale is likewise gainful for overseeing cholesterol. Kale can likewise assist with overseeing circulatory strain because of its undeniable degrees of magnesium and potassium.

Artichokes

Offer your liver a reprieve! Artichokes give a wide assortment of supplements for your blood and liver. Two phytonutrients found in artichokes help the liver produce bile, which is significant in processing fats.

Collard Greens

Collard greens are wealthy in Sulphur-containing intensifies that help your body's detoxification interaction. In addition to the fact that they are high in nutrients K and A, yet collard greens may likewise bring down your danger of bosom, colon, and cellular breakdowns in the lungs due to indole-3-carbinol.

Beets

Beets are high-cell reinforcement vegetables that are additionally wealthy in supplements. Beets contain betaine, which helps the liver free itself of poisons, just as a fiber considered gelatin that clears poisons that have been taken out from the liver.

Spinach

Spinach is low in calories, however, loaded with supplements. Spinach contains nutrients A, C, E, and K, just as thiamine, folate, calcium, iron, and magnesium—the rundown goes on! Flavonoids in spinach assist with holding cholesterol back from oxidizing in your body by going about as a cancer prevention agent.

Chapter 7

Normal Misconceptions About Detoxing

Detox that consumes fewer calories is said to take out poisons from your body, further develop wellbeing, and advance weight reduction.

They frequently include intestinal medicines, diuretics, nutrients, minerals, teas, and different food varieties thought to have detoxing properties.

The expression "poison" with regards to detox eats fewer carbs is approximately characterized. It commonly incorporates toxins, engineered synthetic substances, weighty metals, and prepared food varieties — which all contrarily influence wellbeing.

In any case, mainstream detox abstains from food seldom distinguish the particular poisons they mean to eliminate or the system by which they dispense with them.

Also, no proof backings the utilization of these eating regimens for poison disposal or feasible weight reduction.

Your body has an advanced method of dispensing with poisons that includes the liver, kidneys, stomach-related framework, skin, and lungs.

When these organs are solid, can they successfully kill undesirable substances?

In this way, while detox slims down, don't do anything that your body can't normally do all alone; you can upgrade your body's regular detoxification framework.

Outline

While detox eats less and has an alluring allure, your body is entirely prepared to deal with poisons and other undesirable substances.

1. Breaking point Alcohol

Over 90% of liquor is used in your liver.

Liver proteins use liquor to acetaldehyde, a known malignant growth causing synthetic.

Perceiving acetaldehyde as a poison, your liver proselytes it to an innocuous substance called acetic acid derivation, which is subsequently wiped out from your body.

While observational investigations have shown low-to-direct liquor utilization advantageous for heart wellbeing, extreme drinking can cause a heap of medical issues.

Unreasonable drinking can seriously harm your liver capacity by causing fat development, irritation, and scarring.

At the point when this occurs, your liver can't work enough and play out its fundamental undertakings — including separating waste and different poisons from your body.

In that capacity, restricting or avoiding liquor is outstanding amongst other approaches to keep your body's detoxification framework running solid.

Wellbeing specialists prescribe restricting liquor admission to one beverage each day for ladies and two for men. If you presently don't drink, you shouldn't begin with the potential heart benefits of light-to-direct drinking.

2. Zero in on Sleep

Guaranteeing sufficient and quality rest every night is an unquestionable requirement to help your body's wellbeing and regular detoxification framework.

Dozing permits your mind to revamp and re-energize itself, just as eliminate harmful material results that have gathered for the day.

One of those by-products is a protein called beta-amyloid, which adds to Alzheimer's infection.

With lack of sleep, your body doesn't have the opportunity to play out those capacities so that poisons can develop and influence a few parts of wellbeing.

Helpless rest has been connected to short-and long haul wellbeing results, like pressure, tension, hypertension, coronary illness, type 2 diabetes, and stoutness.

It would help if you rested seven to nine hours of the night consistently to advance great wellbeing.

On the off chance that you experience issues remaining or nodding off around evening time, way of life changes like adhering to a rest timetable and restricting blue light — transmitted from cell phones and PC screens — preceding bed are helpful for further developing rest.

Rundown

Sufficient rest permits your mind to revamp, re-energize, and dispose of poisons that gather for the day.

3. Drink More Water

Water accomplishes such a great deal more than extinguish your thirst. It manages your internal heat level, greases up joints, helps process and supplement retention, and detoxifies your body by eliminating side effects.

Your body's cells should consistently be fixed to work ideally and separate supplements for your body to use as energy.

In any case, these cycles discharge squanders — as urea and carbon dioxide — which cause hurt whenever permitted to develop in your blood.

Water ships these side-effects, proficiently eliminating them through pee, breathing, or sweating. So remaining appropriately hydrated is significant for detoxification.

The excellent day-by-day admission for water is 125 ounces (3.7 liters) for men and 91 ounces (2.7 liters) for ladies. You may require pretty much relying upon your eating regimen, where you live, and your movement level.

Synopsis

Notwithstanding its numerous jobs in your body, water permits your body's detoxification framework to eliminate byproducts from your blood.

To assist you with making your best supper plan, we'll send you master, proof put together direction concerning nourishment and weight reduction.

4. Lessen Your Intake of Sugar and Processed Foods

Sugar and prepared food varieties are believed to be at the base of the present general wellbeing emergencies.

Maximum usage of sweet and exceptionally handled food varieties has been connected to weight and other constant illnesses, like coronary illness, malignancy, and diabetes.

These infections prevent your body's capacity to normally detoxify itself by hurting organs that assume a significant part, like your liver and kidneys.

For instance, intense usage of sweet drinks can cause greasy liver, a condition that adversely impacts liver capacity.

By devouring less low-quality nourishment, you can keep your body's detoxification framework sound.

You can restrict low-quality nourishment by leaving it on the store rack. Not having it in your kitchen removes the enticement through and through.

Supplanting shoddy nourishment with better decisions like foods grown from the ground is likewise a sound method to diminish utilization.

Synopsis

Overabundance lousy nourishment utilization is connected to persistent infections like heftiness and diabetes. These conditions can make hurt organs critical to detoxifying, like your liver and kidneys.

5. Eat Antioxidant-Rich Foods

Cancer prevention agents ensure your phones against harm brought about by particles called free revolutionaries. Oxidative pressure is a condition brought about by the excessive creation of free revolutionaries.

Your body typically delivers these atoms for cell measures, like assimilation. Nonetheless, liquor, tobacco smoke, a horrible eating routine, and openness to toxins can create unreasonable free extremists.

By harming your body's cells, these particles have been embroiled in various conditions, like dementia, coronary illness, liver sickness, asthma, and specific kinds of malignancy.

Eating a routine eating wealthy in cell reinforcements can help your body battle oxidative pressure brought about by overabundance-free revolutionaries and different poisons that expand your danger of sickness.

Zero in on getting cancer prevention agents from food and not supplements, which may, indeed, increment your danger of specific sicknesses when taken in huge sums

Instances of cancer prevention agents incorporate nutrient A, nutrient C, nutrient E, selenium, lycopene, lutein, and zeaxanthin.

Berries, natural products, nuts, cocoa, vegetables, flavors, and drinks like espresso and green tea have the absolute most noteworthy measures of cancer prevention agents.

Synopsis

Devouring an eating regimen wealthy in cancer prevention agents assists your body with diminishing harm brought about by free extremists. It may bring down the danger of infections that can affect detoxification.

6. Eat Foods High in Prebiotics

Gut wellbeing is significant for keeping your detoxification framework sound. Your intestinal cells have a detoxification and discharge framework that shields your gut and body from unsafe poisons, like synthetics.

Great gut wellbeing begins with prebiotics, a sort of fiber that takes care of the great microscopic organisms in your gut called probiotics. With prebiotics, your great microscopic organisms can create supplements called short-chain unsaturated fats that are gainful for the well-being.

The great microscopic organisms in your gut can become unequal with terrible microbes from the utilization of anti-infection agents, helpless dental cleanliness, and diet quality.

Therefore, this undesirable change in microscopic organisms can debilitate your safe and detoxification frameworks and increment your danger of illness and aggravation.

Eating food varieties rich in prebiotics can keep your invulnerable and detoxification frameworks sound. Great food wellsprings of prebiotics incorporate tomatoes, artichokes, bananas, asparagus, onions, garlic, and oats.

7. Lessening Your Salt Intake

For specific individuals, detoxing is a method for killing the overabundance of water.

Burning through a lot of salt can make your body hold overabundance liquid, particularly if you have a condition that influences your kidneys or liver — or on the other hand, on the off chance that you don't drink sufficient water.

This abundance of liquid development can cause swelling and make clothing awkward. If you end up devouring an excessive amount of salt, you can detox yourself of the additional water weight.

While it might sound strange, expanding your water admission is a standout amongst other approaches to kill abundance water weight from burning through an excessive amount of salt.

That is because when you devour an excessive amount of salt and insufficient water, your body delivers an antidiuretic chemical that keeps you from peeing — and like this detoxifying.

By expanding your water admission, your body lessens the discharge of the antidiuretic chemical and builds pee, taking out more water and side effects.

Expanding your admission of potassium-rich food varieties — which offsets sodium's belongings — additionally makes a difference. Food sources wealthy in potassium incorporate potatoes, squash, kidney beans, bananas, and spinach.

Synopsis

Burning through an excess of salt can build water maintenance. You can take out abundance water — and squander — by expanding your admission of water and potassium-rich food varieties.

8. Get Active

Standard exercise — paying little mind to body weight — is related to more extended life and a diminished danger of numerous conditions and illnesses, including type 2 diabetes, coronary illness, hypertension, and certain tumors.

While there are a few instruments behind the medical advantages of activity, decreased aggravation is a central issue.

While some irritation is fundamental for recuperating from contamination or mending wounds, a lot of it debilitates your body's frameworks and advances sickness.

Exercise can help your body's frameworks — including its detoxification framework — work appropriately and secure against sickness by lessening aggravation.

It's suggested that you do no less than 150–300 minutes per seven-day stretch of moderate-force workout — like lively strolling — or 75–150 minutes per seven-day stretch of overwhelming power actual work — like running.

Outline

Ordinary actual work brings down aggravation and permits your body's detoxification framework to work appropriately.

9. Other Helpful Detox Tips

Albeit no current proof backings the utilization of detox eats fewer carbs for eliminating poisons from your body, specific dietary changes and way of life practices may assist with decreasing poison burden and backing your body's detoxification framework.

Eat sulfur-containing food sources. Food sources high in sulfur, like onions, broccoli, and garlic, improve the discharge of substantial metals like cadmium.

Evaluate chlorella. Chlorella is a green growth that has numerous wholesome advantages and may improve the disposal of poisons like substantial metals, as indicated by creature contemplates.

Flavor dishes with cilantro. Cilantro upgrades discharge of specific poisons, for example, hefty metals like lead, and synthetic compounds, including phthalates and insect poisons.

Backing glutathione. Eating sulfur-rich food sources like eggs, broccoli, and garlic helps improve the capacity of glutathione, a significant cancer prevention agent created by your body that is vigorously engaged with detoxification.

Change to average cleaning items. Picking everyday cleaning items like vinegar and heating soft drinks over business cleaning specialists can decrease your openness to poisonous synthetic compounds.

Pick ordinary body care. Utilizing regular antiperspirants, cosmetics, creams, shampoos, and other individual consideration items can likewise lessen your openness to synthetic compounds.

While promising, a considerable lot of these impacts have just been displayed in creature contemplates. In this manner, concentrates on people are expected to affirm these discoveries.

Synopsis

Some way of life and dietary changes may improve your body's regular detoxification framework.

The Bottom Line

Detox tallies calories are said to kill harms, subsequently further creating wellbeing that said, you can upgrade your body's regular detoxification framework and work on your general wellbeing by remaining hydrated, devouring less salt, getting dynamic, and following a cell reinforcement rich eating routine.

www.ingramcontent.com/pod-product-compliance
Ingram Content Group UK Ltd.
Pitfield, Milton Keynes, MK11 3LW, UK
UKHW022009190726
13853UKWH00004B/1823

9 798450 522425